My Journey With Epilepsy

PORTIA HIBBERT

WOODBRIDGE
PUBLISHERS

ISBN (Paperback) 978-1-80704-372-8
ISBN (Hardback) 978-1-80704-373-5
ISBN (eBook) 978-1-80704-374-2

Cover Design by Woodbridge Publishers.

Find out more about our upcoming releases and authors at www.woodbridgepublishers.com and sign up for our newsletter to stay updated!

I'd like to dedicate this book to all those with epilepsy and to those who care for us. Without a good support system, life with epilepsy would be much harder –

Thank you for being there.

TABLE OF CONTENTS

PROLOGUE

Everyone's experience with epilepsy is unique.

Some have the condition. Some may care for someone with epilepsy. Some may know someone with epilepsy. Others may have little to no experience or knowledge of the condition. Those in the same situation will still have their own relationship and experience with it.

An epilepsy diagnosis can happen at any time in a person's life, and there are different diagnoses and types of epilepsy.

This can be from birth or due to any trauma caused later in life, with many different triggers for a seizure.

Treatment plans can vary and evolve throughout a person's life.

The gender of the person impacts all areas of epilepsy: the treatment plan, the hormonal impact, and pregnancy considerations.

While many with epilepsy may find similarities between their experience with epilepsy and mine, there are also vast differences. I don't claim to speak for everyone affected by epilepsy.

This is my journey with epilepsy.

My goal with this book is to grow awareness around epilepsy and help others who are impacted by the condition feel less alone. It is not a well-understood condition, with many knowing only about tonic-clonic seizures and not all the other impacts of epilepsy.

As a 33-year-old, if I look back at my epilepsy over the years, I am amazed at how many changes I have had to adapt to. Having epilepsy is a balance between living, enjoying life, and managing the impacts of having epilepsy.

A bit about myself and my condition before I delve into further detail.

I live in England and was diagnosed with epilepsy 20 years ago. My current diagnosis is genetic generalised epilepsy, and I have both absence and tonic-clonic seizures. I have been on medication since the age of about 19.

My last tonic-clonic seizure was in December 2025, and I currently experience frequent absence seizures.

2025 has been all about changing my medication. I have altered my medications a few times in my life, but this one has had the biggest impact. Perhaps this is due to being older, causing my body and brain to take longer to adjust. It is hard to tell whether it is due to age or due to the many seizures I have had over the years and their long-term impact on my brain. This latest medication change began in December 2024, and I have only just completed the change, with my brain now adjusting to the new medications. Epilepsy has therefore become a much more dominant part of my life - my being - than it ever had before. My triggers are stress and tiredness, though my epilepsy is also aggravated by hayfever, being ill, on my period, in loud white noise environments, and drinking alcohol. I no longer drink alcohol, a decision made because of my epilepsy.

Since 2021, I've noticed increased memory impairment, slower brain processing, and difficulty focusing. These issues have steadily worsened over the years, becoming a greater concern since 2023.

In this book, my memories will differ depending on how far back I am going. Although I will try to recall as much as possible and maintain consistency, I apologise that some areas will lack detail or even differ slightly from those who were present! I include them to share their impact as they remain important parts of my journey.

My journey with epilepsy is a constantly evolving path. My relationship with the condition has altered over the years, as has the severity of the seizures I have had.

DIAGNOSIS

When I was 14, my mum took me to the paediatrician. She took the lead during these appointments due to my age. Although I remember my doctor, who was very kind and reassuring, the exact process is somewhat hazy. I cannot remember the exact trigger point for my referral to neurology; however, I do know that I had been having moments of hesitation, often during conversations. To determine the root cause of these hesitant moments, I needed to have some tests. My doctor wanted to see one of these hesitation moments on camera, so that he had a visual example to work from. Alongside this, I was booked in for both an MRI and an EEG. An EEG (electroencephalogram) is a test that measures the electrical activity of the brain. Once the results of these had been collected, they would be able to make a diagnosis and provide some answers.

I come from a loud family. We all talk over each other, always have done, and conversation can become a jumble of voices. A lovely family environment, but apparently too much for my brain to handle! I seemed more prone to these blanks, or "absence seizures" as we now know them to be, at the end of a school day when we were all eating supper together. So, during supper was when we tried to capture me having an absence seizure.

At this time in my life, I had braces and disliked people watching me eat, so having a camera pointed at me throughout supper was horrible - I really hated it! In my mind, we had this camera pointing at me for at least a week of mealtimes after school, but I am told that it was only once...I have no proof either way, so happy to accept the latter as fact. If it was only once, then it seared into my mind. Like I said, I hated it. We were "successful" in capturing an absence on film, which was the first time I saw myself having these episodes, and I remember feeling pretty emotional about it. A success - we had captured it - but it was evidence that there *was* something wrong, which was upsetting to see and realise. However, we had some evidence for my paediatrician to work with. Homework complete.

I had the MRI, which was loud and a little claustrophobic, but the technicians played me some Disney music during the scan, which helped. I was not allowed to see my brain scan, though I was curious as to what it looked like – it was going to the specialist for interpretation - but I always wish I had a copy of my MRI scans, even if I cannot understand them. It would be great to see the comparison of my brain over the years.

My EEG was up next in the path towards a diagnosis. I remember sitting in this room at Furness General Hospital with a very kind male specialist attaching a load of wires to my brain with a Vaseline-type paste - it was quite a weird feeling, but not at all painful. To clarify, they are just stuck to your scalp - nothing attached internally!

Whilst my brain activity was being recorded, I went through different activities. I was asked to hyperventilate, stare at a light which flashed at different speeds, leading to a strobe effect, open and close my eyes at certain points, and then to rest and try to sleep for about 20 minutes.

This whole process exhausted my brain, and the hyperventilating in particular did not make me feel good - this was the part of the test that ended up inducing epileptic brain activity. The flashing lights did not result in epileptic brain activity, but I did find it draining. It is a common thought that people with epilepsy are triggered by flashing lights; however, only about 5% of people with epilepsy are photosensitive. There are many, more common, triggers.

The specialist kindly removed the wires from my head and brushed the paste out. My hair just looked super greasy. After an hour or so of the EEG test, the results were sent to the specialist to be read alongside my MRI scan and the video I had provided.

I was diagnosed with juvenile generalised epilepsy, experiencing absence seizures. At this early point, due to the video capturing my absence, we knew that tiredness and auditory overstimulation could induce my seizures.

Since becoming an adult, my diagnosis changed to genetic generalised epilepsy, experiencing both absence and tonic-clonic seizures. My diagnosis is "generalised epilepsy" because the seizures affect both sides of the brain, and the epileptic activity is coming from multiple areas of the brain. I equate this to having a lightning storm occur throughout the brain when I have a seizure.

DENIAL

I didn't tell anyone that I had epilepsy. I wouldn't let my family talk to people about it and have always hated being referred to as epileptic (this part has not changed).

I was in full-blown denial, feeling embarrassed and ashamed of having epilepsy. I didn't want people to judge me because of my epilepsy and know me as "the girl with epilepsy."

I did not want it to define me.

Throughout my teens, I had absence seizures, and they have evolved throughout my life. Pre-diagnosis and the first year of my diagnosis, my absence seizures presented themselves as moments of hesitation, mainly mid-conversation. They lasted seconds, sometimes even less, but they became increasingly intense. I would not be able to remember what I was talking about or what the person I was talking to was saying. I would be physically standing, but mentally, my brain checked out.

My experience of them intensified from an episode that was not completely blank to me to being visual blackouts, which were even harder to come back from. Looking back, there was a correlation between these changes and hormonal changes.

I would come around to comments that referred to my lack of response to a comment or question or to a remark about my facial expression. My face would have slackened, emotionless, like giving evils.

I tried to mask my episodes as much as possible. I would apologise and try to continue the conversation.

Aged 15, I told my best friend at the time about my seizures. I cannot remember her response, but whatever it was did not change my feelings of shame or embarrassment, which kept me from telling others. Not her fault by any means, but it was just too big a thing to get over at that age. As a teenager, there is so much to label you as "other" and no one needed additional ammunition.

Growing up, technology was a much smaller part of our lives than it is now, and so, more easily restricted. In my family, we had certain ages when we would be allowed things like a phone or a laptop. At 15, we got our own laptop; before this, we had our family computer. The big windows computer, huge monitor. We were each allowed 30 minutes a day on it. There was always an argument when our 30 minutes were up, and it was my brother or sister's turn! Of course, we all tried to extend our turn for as long as possible.

Before I had reached the age to get a phone, a friend lent me her old phone to use until I was old enough to have my own. I thought I was super smart, but then my parents found out, and I had to give the phone back. Back then, those limits on technology were easier to maintain—and far healthier for the brain.

When I got a laptop, it was so liberating. It was the era of Myspace, Bebo, the start of Facebook, and MSN Messenger. There were increasing amounts of technological distractions. I just wanted to stay up late talking to friends. This overpowered the need to look after myself and manage my epilepsy; I didn't want to acknowledge I had epilepsy.

With the increasing presence of technology, plus being a slightly defiant teenager, it got to the point where my laptop and phone had to be left downstairs at night. Best for me and my health, but as a teenager, it was not a welcome restriction!

It was easy to stay in denial. I wasn't having tonic-clonic seizures, and though my absences were tough, they generally only occurred when stressed or tired. Plus, they were subtle enough to try to hide, something I felt I was becoming good at.

I went to parties and drank alcohol, pushing my brain and testing my alcohol tolerance with enthusiasm.

My absences began to follow a clearer pattern. After late nights, especially if I had been drinking, I would often wake up and immediately slip into a cluster of absences. On the worst days, the moment I opened my eyes, my brain felt overwhelmed, and I had to return to bed to give myself more rest.

MEDICATIONS

My epilepsy has changed since diagnosis. It is almost impossible to determine if these changes are due to medication side effects, the medication altering my epilepsy, hormones, or changes in my brain.

Over the years, my brain has been struck by the many lightning storms of my seizures. As someone with generalised epilepsy, the storm hits many areas of the brain, impacting many different cognitive areas over time. Also, over time, the brain matures, and by around 25, it has developed. To separate the brain from the epilepsy and medication is nearly impossible. Who would I have been without epilepsy? Are the changes that I experience just characteristics of my personality or the impact of having epilepsy? There is so much unknown about the brain and epilepsy, so it is hard to have clear answers.

The main priority of the neurologist when finding a suitable treatment plan is to manage the tonic-clonic seizures, as they are the most dangerous and can be fatal. Medication is chosen depending on your type of seizure, type of epilepsy (focal or generalised), with other considerations to factor in, such as gender. As a woman with genetic generalised epilepsy, who has both absence and tonic-clonic seizures, not all treatment plans are open to me. Surgery, for example, is not an option to me as my epilepsy does not occur in a specific part of my brain. Anti-seizure medications have their different strengths and focus areas, some of which would not help with my type of epilepsy. Some help manage tonic-clonics, some help with absence seizures, and everyone reacts differently to them.

Before starting any medication, we tried to manage my epilepsy with acupuncture. Whilst I was only having absence seizures, and along with my neurologist, wanted to avoid medication for as long as possible, we looked for alternative options. My Dad would take me to an acupuncturist, who would treat me and suggest supplements or foods to take or avoid to help with my seizures. After the treatment, I would leave with a plaster on my neck, which had a tiny needle in it, like a very tiny drawing pin. It didn't hurt, but tried to help with brain tension, and I left it in as long as possible. I am sure this helped in some ways, but it did not remove the eventual requirement for Western medication.

The first medication I was on was Lamotrigine. I started at a low dose, slowly increasing to a higher dose as required. When it was clear that they were not stopping the tonic-clonic seizures, I added Levetiracetam or Keppra, which is the brand name.

I came off Lamotrigine and remained on Keppra, increasing to 4 grams a day, the maximum dose. There is something called "Keppra rage," which is a common side effect of the drug that can manifest in different ways. To me, it is like having a cinder block on my emotions; all my emotions are dulled. If I am feeling down, I can feel depressed. Happy emotions and excitement are lessened. By 2014, my lower mood was noticed by close friends. Though I felt this side effect, I didn't know how obvious it had become to others. Taking this amount of Keppra led to me also being diagnosed with depression. Along with my mood change, I was still having tonic-clonic seizures fairly frequently; it was clear Keppra was not right for me.

At the age of 22, I started Sodium Valproate, the brand name of Epilim. As a sexually active woman, Sodium Valproate is a tough one to be prescribed and is not recommended unless you are very careful. I was not planning on having children any time soon, but had to take folic acid alongside the Epilim to reduce any risks to the foetus if I accidentally fell pregnant. Sodium Valproate increases birth risks from 2-3% (average healthy woman) to 10-13%; this figure is even higher when looking at the risks of causing neurological specific disorders. This is a female-specific risk to consider, and in every doctor's appointment, I was reminded of these risks. For both genders, however, there is also the risk of reduced fertility from this medication. If I were a man, this could have been a potential long-term medication for me. It ended up working fairly well to control my seizures, making my epilepsy more manageable, and I experienced very few side effects whilst on it.

Stress is one of my triggers. It is something I have to keep in check, though at times this is hard to do, especially if life or work becomes stressful. Aside from potentially inducing a migraine, I used to get really bad nosebleeds. They became so bad that in 2015, when I was working in recruitment in Czechia, our HR manager had to take me to get my nose cauterised. Quite an amusingly daunting situation of going into a tiled room with my HR manager and two doctors who only spoke Czech. I had to trust the HR manager to translate for me, so I knew what was going on. It ended up all fine, and the procedure was a success.

My stress nose bleeds decreased, but from 2016, I was having to take a prescribed amount of aspirin for my migraines. Related to my epilepsy, I have suffered from migraines as long as I can remember. Before my epilepsy diagnosis, my migraines would always be very intense, and I would often be sick as a result. During my first job in London, due to my triggers of stress and lack of sleep, I would often experience migraines that would last 2 weeks. These would also often come with an increased amount of absence seizures. This happened frequently enough that by 2018, I needed to be referred to a migraine specialist. I was eventually put on Propranolol, a medication that targets migraines, and this has made a huge improvement. I am still on Propranolol, and since being on my current dose, I have stopped having the ridiculously long migraines that were really debilitating. When they crop up now, they are a tell that I am or have been stressed about something. However, they are manageable, less frequent, and don't last as long as they used to, which is a win. Migraines are often dismissed as headaches, but the pain, nausea, and inability to function normally should not be underestimated.

Once I was in a long-term relationship, I decided to change my medication. I planned to one day have children, and, in the meantime, I did not like the increased risk that Sodium Valproate would have on the foetus if I were to fall pregnant. It was time to change and find a medication that was a healthier option in the event of a pregnancy. This process of changing a medication takes time, with potential trial and error as the medication or dosage may end up not working for the patient.

Late 2018 to 2019, I started on Zonisamide, a medication that was safer to have children on than Sodium Valproate. Sodium Valproate had also not been completely successful in managing my seizures. Whilst taking it, I would still have tonic-clonic seizures but with a more predictable pattern. However, I was also still going out late and drinking alcohol, which increased my risk of seizures as I would push my body and sleep poorly. The new medication, Zonisamide, made my seizures even more predictable in nature, solidifying a behaviour pattern. I wouldn't have absence seizures randomly, only after a late night, and generally as a warning before a tonic-clonic seizure. I had more confidence in their predictability and my brain's day-to-day capabilities.

My last tonic-clonic seizure for a long time was in January 2019. I was drinking increasingly less alcohol and finally taking on board the doctor's frequent suggestion to go alcohol free.

Zonisamide was a massive help in managing my tonic-clonic seizures. Throughout my time taking Zonisamide, I only had one tonic-clonic seizure, and that was right at the start as I adjusted to it. But I had also stopped drinking. Removing alcohol enabled me to notice my natural tiredness levels better and helped to improve my sleep efficiency. The days when I would have been hungover and sleep-deprived became days to manage only the sleep deprivation from the night before. I continued to experience stress, and migraines would flare up every now and then, but the Propranolol kept them from becoming too intrusive or causing seizures.

In 2022, I was still having absence seizures whilst taking just the Zonisamide, so my neurologist and I decided to introduce another medication alongside it - Ethosuximide, otherwise known by the brand name, Epesri. It is not as common a medication, and so since late 2022, whilst I was taking Ethosuximide, it would sometimes become hard to order from the pharmacy. Possible, but as a more expensive medication, the pharmacy would only order it in when requested. They wouldn't hold it in stock, and sometimes their supplier would even be out of the medication. I had to be on the ball and order it with more time for the GP and pharmacy to process the request.

Once, I had put the prescription request in, well enough in advance, before I went on holiday. By the time I went to collect my medications and discovered it was not there, it was too late for it to come in before I went away. As many pharmacies don't hold it in stock, it took a while to figure out a plan to get hold of the medication. I had to coordinate with my sister, who would be in London before joining me on holiday. My pharmacy was able to send the script to a London pharmacy, which rushed it, enabling my sister to go collect it on her lunch break before joining me in Italy. Thank you, Olivia!

For a while, this cocktail of Zonisamide, Epesri, and Propranolol was keeping my migraines and both seizure types at bay. However, my brain was struggling, increasingly so, with memory recall, auditory processing, and general fatigue. It was also impacting my performance at work.

Then, new research came to me from my neurologist that Zonisamide was no longer recommended to women who wanted to conceive. Though I did not have a partner, as previously mentioned, it can take a while to change and settle into a new medication. In my experience, changes of medication to enable someone to safely get pregnant tend to be suggested *as* you are looking to conceive. To me, this makes little sense as it can take many months to change medication. It would require further planning and a potential delay in conceiving. It, of course, depends on the type of epilepsy and its intensity, but in my situation, I prefer to be ready for when I want children. So, I prepared my body yet again for a medication change.

The risk in different medications can be due to how the medication is ingested and helps to form the baby, increasing risks such as abnormalities and defects, but there is also an impact on breastfeeding. Some medications can come out through breast milk, and others don't. The ideal is, of course, not to feed your baby contaminated breast milk.

It was decided that in December 2024, I would begin my 14-week schedule away from Zonisamide and Ethosuximide. In the November prior to the change, I had a large cluster of absences, which was further confirmation that these medications were no longer effective, and the decision to change them was the right one. When my body is in this state of having multiple absence seizures, it is like it is slowly shutting down. My core gets cold, and I feel jittery as more energy goes into my brain just functioning. When I reach this point, it is hard to calm my brain down when I try to go to sleep. To help with this, I have a rescue medication called Clobazam.

The evening in November 2024 confirmed that changing my medication was the right thing to do. Although I wasn't having tonic-clonic seizures, I was having fairly frequent absences, often in the evening when tired, but they could begin as early as 8 pm. My medication was also potentially increasing brain fatigue, memory loss, and processing difficulties, side effects that had seeped into my work life. As previously mentioned, it is tough to know whether these were medication side effects or epilepsy side effects – how my brain had developed. I had a set of scans in October 2024, prior to any medication changes, an EEG, and an MRI, and the results showed that there was still "epileptic activity". This activity occurred while on Zonisamide and Ethosuximide. Further proof that the medication wasn't completely effective, so with the medication change, I had hope that I would see improvements in my epilepsy and the side effects. I include some photos here of me during this EEG to give you an idea of the procedure.

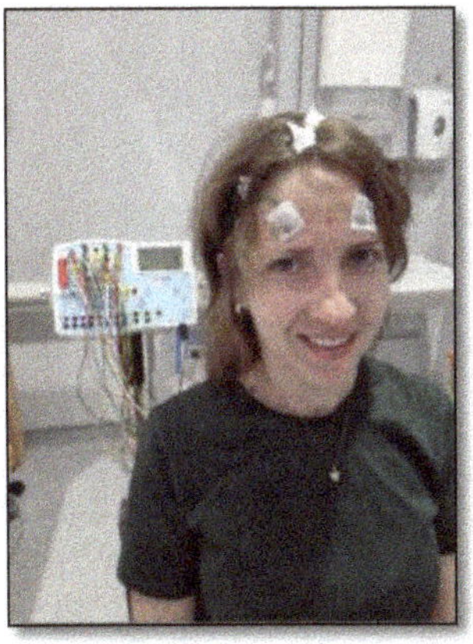 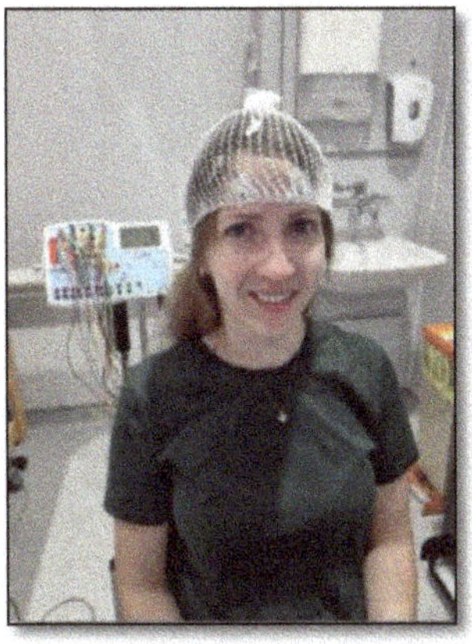

So, I was to change medication. The two medication options available to me, a woman with absence and tonic-clonic seizures, who wanted to conceive, were Keppra (Levetiracetam) and Lamotrigine. I had already been on both medications when I was younger, so having to return to something I had already tried was frustrating. I had changed away from them previously because I had continued to experience seizures whilst on both, when taken separately and together. I reassured myself that my brain was different now, it was fully developed, and I no longer drink alcohol - the conditions had changed.

My neurologist and I decided to change to Keppra first, as it had a shorter titration schedule than Lamotrigine. By this, I mean it takes a shorter amount of time to move onto the goal dosage of medication. If it didn't work, then we would try Lamotrigine. The plan was to reduce and come off Zonisamide, add in Keppra, and then reduce and come off Ethosuximide, then see how I was doing. Adjustments to the dosage were made each week.

I moved onto the agreed amount of Keppra over the weeks, and I really struggled. My brain was trying to compensate for the lack of support it had received from Zonisamide and Epesri. My brain was so tired. Once on Keppra, I needed to sleep more; everything was an effort, and pushing myself to exhaustion could be dangerous. I had an increasing number of absence seizures. But happily, the medication change to Keppra did not induce a tonic-clonic seizure. Within about 1 month of being on the agreed amount of Keppra, after the 14 weeks of change, it was clear I needed to further increase my dosage. This didn't sit well with me, having previously experienced the emotional lows of Keppra. Regardless, I increased to 1500mg bi-daily - in the morning and evening. Eventually, small improvements in my capabilities and brain power were evident, but I was still not fully recovered. I was exhausted and having multiple absences a week.

Since taking Keppra, aside from experiencing lower and dulled emotions, I need much more sleep and have also gained weight. I find it harder to know my body's needs compared to when I was on Zonisamide and Ethosuximide. Before, what I ate, how I felt, and my body weight would all relate to each other and be more manageable. Now, it is not so clear what the correlation is. The weight gain is not related to food input; the body is harder to understand, predict, and manage.

By mid-2025, it had been over 6 years since my last tonic-clonic seizure. But I could not go one week without an absence seizure.

Once it was clear that Keppra alone was not working, my neurologist and I decided to add in Lamotrigine, an addition that would take many weeks. I have now finally completed this change and am currently waiting for my brain to adjust to the final dosage and mix of Lamotrigine, Levetiracetam (Keppra), and Propranolol.

For many years, I have also had the aforementioned rescue medication, Clobazam. I typically use it if I cannot sleep and need to relax my brain, but I can also take it if I am experiencing absences.

Taking multiple medications twice a day also comes with some admin work! Aside from ordering the medication, I have to sort out my medication, which takes some time. A few years ago, I gave in and purchased a pill box, which I later added to so that I could prepare two weeks of medication at a time - a life changer! I will say, I am forever grateful that those with epilepsy are exempt from paying NHS prescription fees. I would be much poorer if I had to pay for the multiple prescriptions I have to take in order to live with reduced seizures. I fear that without this, many people would opt out of taking their medication, as it would just be too expensive.

Having epilepsy is a constant balance of checking in with your brain and distinguishing between the controllable and uncontrollable. The things we're familiar with naturally change over the course of our lives. As we get older, our bodies react differently than they did when we were younger; we bounce back slower. When you have a long-term condition such as epilepsy, there are many aspects that you cannot control, so it is important to focus on what you can control. If I get ill, with the flu or virus, I take longer to recover as my brain then requires additional energy. The energy that also goes into getting over a bug can reduce my brain's focus on managing my epilepsy, so often seizures are more readily induced. I cannot change that my brain is to some extent "my weak spot" and is always affected by an illness. But I can change some things. The decision of stopped drinking helped me recognise my limits and manage fatigue more effectively. Sometimes medication induces weight gain; this can sometimes be regulated by diet and exercise, sometimes it can't. Although we cannot control the parts of the brain affected by epilepsy, we can learn how the brain influences other areas of the body and take steps to reduce the impact of our condition. Paying attention to nutrition or using appropriate supplements may support overall brain function and cognitive recovery. For example, I recently noticed that my epilepsy gets worse when I am on my period, a condition known as catamenial epilepsy. Until 2025, I had not recognised this pattern, but now I am aware it makes so much sense when I look back at previous seizure patterns. When I am on my period, I try to be more aware of the food I am eating and making sure I get enough of what my body needs.

With these latest medications, I still see side effects, though the seizures seem to be reducing week by week, which is promising. I am still working with the side effects of memory loss, less clear or foggy days, harder to control weight, but most of all, a greater requirement for sleep. I have to have a good night's sleep for about 10 hours a night to be able to function the next day. This fatigue interrupts the weekly structure hugely. Those who also have this as a side effect will find it harder to commit to a normal work week and allow their days to be consistently busy. The idea of living as I used to, with a full week of a 9 am-5/6 pm job and social commitments, seems so far away to me.

A big lesson I have learned throughout years of medical appointments and treatment plan discussions is that I am the expert of my brain. Do your research, come to the specialist with suggestions, and get to know your body. For these appointments and general tracking of seizures, I have found using an epilepsy journal app to be a huge help. You can note patterns over time by recording medications and seizures, which can all be sent to your neurologist. I only wish I had used something similar earlier on! You know your condition best, so use the professionals for advice and medical support.

MY SEIZURES

I tend to only have absence and tonic-clonic seizures. However, I have also had one partial seizure.

Absence seizures are brief moments of hesitation or staring; a few seconds where your brain "glitches". You lose awareness, but it is short enough that your body continues to function, for example, you stay sitting or standing.

A partial seizure is when you remain aware and conscious, but the brain is having a moment, a glitch, which you have little to no control over. For the one time I had a partial seizure, I was having breakfast in the kitchen at university. I was in the middle of putting the spoon to my mouth, and my hand froze, I made a noise, and my head kept ticking to the right. I had no control over this action but was aware of what was happening.

A tonic-clonic seizure is a full-body jerking and stiffening of the body. There are two phases to this seizure. In the "tonic" phase, the muscles and body stiffen; during the "clonic" phase, the body jerks and moves about. There is a loss of consciousness followed by the stiffening then jerking of the muscles. During these seizures, there can be teeth grinding, noises, biting your tongue or cheek, and loss of bladder control.

There are many further types of seizure, which I do not experience and so cannot speak to. Seizures generally fall into either generalised seizures, which I have, or focal seizures, which come from specific areas of the brain. Diagnoses can change over time, and people can experience a variety of seizures, which can vary in frequency, length, and intensity.

ABSENCE SEIZURES

Often taken for daydreaming or hesitation in thought, an absence seizure is a blip - a stop-and-stare moment. You lose awareness, but potentially only for a couple of seconds.

When I first had absence seizures in my teens, they were super intense. More of a blackout, but my physical state would be in autopilot. My brain would be out, but my body stays standing. My face would therefore go blank, and I would look like I was giving evils as I'd have dead eyes.

Over time, the intensity of these changed. Whether they changed in nature or I just handled them better, I am not too sure. I think probably a bit of both.

The body is an amazing thing. During absences, the body can react faster than the brain. When I was about fifteen, I went on holiday to France with my family and experienced my first real scare with these absences. I was sitting, or rather balancing, on a bike barrier at the start of a bridge when an absence came over me. My body suddenly slackened, and I fell backwards, but I managed to catch myself on the other side of the barrier just behind me. The speed at which my body reacted and returned from the absence was incredible, even though my mind took longer to fully come back. It was frightening, yet also an impressive example of how differently the body and brain respond during these absences. They happen so quickly, but they can feel longer and more intense from the inside than they appear on the outside.

I would have absences frequently enough that I learned to deal with them. I could pick up with the conversation and quickly hide it with an "I've lost my train of thought" or "what was I saying again?" often apologising. I resumed in autopilot and wasn't too bothered by them; I just wanted to cover them up.

Even with the masking, I always felt embarrassed, sometimes had a painful headache, and mainly, I had no idea what had been going on pre-seizure. I had to catch up fast.

They used to only come in the morning if I had an inefficient night's sleep, sometimes exacerbated by drinking alcohol.

Because of the frequency, I had never counted the gap between my absence seizures, which I was able to do with tonic-clonics.

But suddenly it had been a month since my last absence.

And then two months.

I managed to have a year free from all seizures, absences, and tonic-clonics, from December 2021 to the start of 2023. The absences can sometimes be so hard to detect. The difference between being lost in thought and having an absence is the feeling the absences come with. Easy for others to ignore, but I was unconscious, and my brain was glitching, so it comes with a certain feeling. The first one I had, after a year without them, was gutting. Though I still didn't quite have faith in my brain to be able to start driving, with the multitasking and ability to take in all potential hazards, I was at least at a point where I *could* apply for a driving license if I wanted to. But now, in a second, the clock had reset.

I continued to have absences infrequently enough, perhaps once a month, but with a new pattern of evening tiredness being a greater trigger. Since being a teenager, they had mainly occurred in the mornings. But since my latest medication change to Epesri, I could be triggered by an overstimulating environment in the evening, like a pub or dinner party. My brain would get overstimulated and just check out, and it would become harder to focus on speaking and engaging in a conversation with people. In November 2024, when I was at a Halloween party at a friend's house, I had at least 10 intense absences in quick succession. In the middle of talking to someone, I had an intense absence for a few seconds, and within about another minute, I was gone again. I was taking a picture of some friends when I realised I was just standing there with the phone up in the air, not taking any photos! They were all smiling, picture ready, and had no idea I hadn't yet taken any photos! Fairly amusing, and I did eventually get a picture of them, but I realised I had to say goodbye and leave pretty quickly. As I said bye to my hosts, I continued to have intense absences, making my exit rather slow. My body went into autopilot as I went to say bye to one. I just walked straight past him as I had an absence, then had to come back. These ones did not go unnoticed. I managed to get in a taxi and felt a little better as I relaxed for the journey and didn't have the noise of people chatting or a conversation to focus on. After an evening like this, my focus is on avoiding a tonic-clonic seizure, but my mind is in overdrive. In these situations, I have to take Clobazam to help me get to sleep.

Since embarking on my latest medication change, absences have become the norm, an exhausting part of life. As of November 2025, I was having at least five a week. These may be without trigger, no late night, enough sleep, and no alcohol. The unpredictability is so frustrating. The neurologist and epilepsy nurses are happy that I only had two tonic-clonic seizures since changing the medication, which I am also happy about. However, absence seizures are both knackering and damaging to the brain, impacting your life in other ways that aren't visible. It isn't just having the seizure that impacts you; it is the brain fog and lack of energy that surrounds it. There's also an increased need for sleep to aid recovery and the fatigue that impacts processing and memory recall skills.

I frequently forget words and just have to say one that sounds familiar and has come to mind, with the hope that the person I am speaking with will find the word I was looking for or just understand what I meant anyway.

I have no idea how many absence seizures I have had in my life, but it would be a depressingly high number.

MY FIRST TONIC-CLONIC SEIZURE

The month I turned 18, I had my first tonic-clonic seizure.

The night before, I had been at an 18th birthday party and then slept on the floor of a marquee, along with many other people. In the morning, I woke up after having a very inefficient night's sleep and tried to interact with people, having breakfast and saying goodbye before grabbing a lift back to school with a friend. During these interactions, I was having frequent and intense absences, clusters that increased the more I pushed my brain to function. I managed to get some sleep in the car while my friend drove us back to school. As we were driving through the school, I had my first tonic-clonic seizure.

My friend managed to get me out of the car and onto the ground. I believe I had one mainly in the car, scaring the life out of him, as I don't believe he knew I had epilepsy. Not many people did at this time. I chose a great place to have this seizure, on the cricket pitch in the middle of the school campus, interrupting a cricket match. A fantastically subtle announcement of my epilepsy. I came around very disoriented and lying on the grass, facing my boyfriend at the time, who had been playing cricket (before I stopped the match!)

I felt very nauseous and super confused, and I remember trying to get up and Ben telling me to stay lying down and rest. Coming around to a familiar face and calming voice made me feel safe. This is important as I felt vulnerable, unwell, and in no state to move, so being reassured of your safety makes a huge difference. My body was knackered, all my muscles were shot, and the nausea got the better of me, as it sometimes does after a seizure.

After a minute, I was able to take in my matron, an ambulance parked on the grass near me, and the fact that I had wet myself. I was able to gauge what must have happened, and I burst into tears. I was embarrassed and had lost. The epilepsy had won. This feeling of loss is hard to describe. Up until this point, I had kept the tonic-clonic seizures at bay. The hope is always that the brain will somehow heal itself and you'll grow out of it. This seizure showed that my epilepsy was not improving at all. This was the worst-case scenario; I was now having tonic-clonic seizures, and my epilepsy would be harder to hide.

I woke up again in the hospital, potentially in between as well, though I was not aware. I had familiar faces around me and had been told my mum was on her way, driving down to Shrewsbury from home in the Lake District.

After having a seizure, your mind is not in a strong place. I was emotional, kept crying, and forgetting what had happened. You just want to carry on, but then your body and mind just hurt. You need sleep, and so you drift in and out of it. The doctors ask you seemingly easy questions that are the hardest things to answer, and make your brain hurt.

"Portia, do you know what day it is?" I guess a day - incorrect. Frustration.

"Portia, do you know why you are here?" No. Pain increases - why don't I know? Tears again.

"Portia, do you know who this is?" (Pointing to someone I should know, but whose name I can't think of)

These questions are necessary for a doctor to ask in order to understand the cognitive status, but they feel impossible to answer. Memory has gone, and your brain needs rest and time to recover. My experience is that if you force your brain to do things before it's ready, it is overwhelmed and will divert to having a seizure or become increasingly painful.

I eventually recovered from my seizure and returned to school.

MY SECOND TONIC-CLONIC SEIZURE

In 2011, I went on my gap year, travelling with my friend around Latin America for nearly 5 months. Looking back, I am very thankful that I was not on medication at the time! Having to take 5 months of medication away with me would have taken up my whole bag.

I had still only had the one tonic-clonic by the time we left for Peru; my absences weren't too bad, only presenting themselves when I was overtired or hungover. As had become the case, they tended to occur in the morning if I hadn't had enough sleep. I was able to manage them by going back to bed and not pushing my brain into overdrive.

My friend and I were about 3 months into our trip and staying at a hostel in Guatemala, I believe.

From here, we will enter a period of hazy memories and "as I understand it". But certain details are not so important. Sometimes, if we put too much pressure on ourselves to remember things, it can just be disheartening when we don't get there.

So, we were in Guatemala, partway through our backpacking trip, staying on mattresses in the attic area of a hostel. There were lines of mattresses on each side of the attic. About $5 a night - perfect! We went out with some other travellers, having a late night, and returning to our mattresses upstairs, sharing the space with many other people arriving back at different times, snoring, etc. Safe to say that I did not have a good night's sleep! In the morning,

I was queuing for the shower downstairs. Next thing I know, I am lying on a bed in a shared dorm, with a concerned guy sitting next to me. I was disoriented and had no idea I had had a tonic-clonic seizure or who this person was. It became clear that I was safe, but that I had experienced a seizure. This man was very kind and turned out to be a junior doctor on his travels, and had luckily been in the shower queue at the same time as me. My friend had been with me all morning as I slept and had left me a note to say she'll be back shortly, but understandably had to grab some food. I continued to sleep off my second tonic-clonic seizure, emotional and full of grief, frustration, and shame.

AN ERA OF TONIC-CLONIC SEIZURES

When I returned from my travels just before I turned 19, I knew I needed to go on medication, but I was not yet ready to give up drinking alcohol - I was about to go to University and wanted to fully enjoy my experience there. I began to take my first medication, Lamotrigine, before I started my 4 years at Reading.

My seizures became more predictable in their pattern. If I had a late night and drank alcohol, I was increasingly likely to have to have a rest day the following day. A late night could be going out or socialising with people, and in whatever situation, I was overstimulating my brain. I was pushing it beyond what it could manage, and I ended up suffering for it the next day. If I had a night of insufficient sleep, I would wake up, and the absences would begin. I might be on the way to brushing my teeth and would just stand there confused, or I would walk around aimlessly with my toothbrush. Whenever I didn't listen to the warning of my absences, more would come, and eventually I would have a tonic-clonic seizure.

The only way to avoid a tonic-clonic seizure would be to go back to sleep and allow my brain to recuperate.

Sometimes, if I push my brain too far, it gets agitated, and I find it hard to sleep. It feels weird, and my body has almost started to go into shutdown mode. I get very cold and almost internally fidgety. This still happens to me today, though other aspects have changed. The only way to calm my brain down enough to sleep is to take some Clobazam, which mildly sedates me. Judging when I have had enough sleep is tricky. Sometimes I wake up and still need more, sometimes I try and start my day and about an hour later notice I need more sleep, and other days I wake up rested. This process is frustrating and always comes with a side of FOMO. Often sleeping in the day means I have to miss out on something, and when I am already feeling vulnerable and down about being in a bad way, I feel emotional and sad about missing out. It is often when we feel weak and vulnerable that we are more susceptible to our emotions.

Though it is forever disappointing, the realisation that I have just had a seizure, and perhaps even because of this disappointment, I try and find the funny side in some of my seizures, made easier with hindsight. I also try not to dwell too much on others' experiences of my seizures, as this is a tough pill to swallow. I hate that something that I have done can be a traumatic or upsetting experience for someone.

However, I will share some of my experiences that particularly stand out for various reasons.

Before I went to university, I stayed over at a friend's house with a couple of other friends, drinking wine and hanging out. With the alcohol, conversation late into the night, and an unfamiliar bed, my sleep wasn't fantastic. I woke up too early and went to the loo. I started having multiple absence seizures, and my body went into autopilot. I somehow decided to go get changed in the downstairs bathroom, not the closest one to me. No one else was awake. I ended up taking myself and my clothes downstairs, seeing the old family dog, and heading into the bathroom. It took me a while to head downstairs as I kept having intense absence seizures, stopping, confused, and questioning what I was doing, and then continuing down the stairs.

It's a bit of a blur as I had a couple of tonic-clonic seizures, but I had walked out of the bathroom mid-changing and topless, and then proceeded to have a tonic-clonic seizure in the front hall; my subconscious was perhaps going to alert someone. I was found on the floor not long after my first seizure.

I remember my t-shirt being laid across my chest, the sight of a paramedic having tea with my mum, and the ambulance parked close by. There is nothing much for a paramedic to do other than to sit, wait, and observe as a seizure happens. I took a long time to come around; my mum had been called by my friends, and she finally took me home when I was able to move. I was just so embarrassed; I had had multiple seizures, they had hit me hard, and my body was exhausted. I was still recovering the next day and received a very lovely get-well card from the people I had been with. This sort of kindness makes such a difference and is not to be underestimated.

Embarrassment subsides with time, but back then, having tonic-clonics was a fairly new thing, and the fear of judgment was massive. I can now see this as one of my more amusing seizures. It is also a lesson of how to deal with a seizure. My friends had covered me with my t-shirt to reduce my embarrassment, called for help (my mum) and an ambulance, and I came around to familiarity and calm. Who the ambulance was called by and whether the ambulance was called before or after my second seizure, I have no idea, and isn't particularly relevant here. I was made to feel safe.

Another scary but slightly amusing seizure was whilst at my family home, perhaps during the university holidays. We had been socialising the night before, perhaps a dinner or drinks party, and I was going to take a shower. I locked the bathroom that I shared with my sister and proceeded to have a tonic-clonic seizure, where I damaged my ribs, broke the loo seat, and scared my sister. Olivia heard me fall and make noises, something the body does when seizing, and took ages trying to break into the bathroom, eventually successfully reaching me. This stood out for a few reasons. It was one of the worst in terms of experience for my sister, and an extra painful one for me due to falling on the loo seat with my ribs. They still sometimes hurt today, and at the time, they were especially painful. However, I somehow find some amusement in breaking the loo seat. As a result, I now don't lock bathroom doors unless I am feeling absolutely fine. The danger is very real when you have a tonic-clonic, and the damage done can be lasting.

I have had many tonic-clonics, many, many absence seizures, and one partial seizure. At the time of the partial seizure, I did not notice how unusual this type of seizure was for me.

I am lucky that my tonic-clonic seizures tend to have a warning of absences, but other than that, I have no warning. The absences tend to push me to go back to sleep when possible. However, denial can push you to carry on. A commitment? Can't cancel, it's too late, I'll be okay to push through. Denial enables unwise decisions to be made, putting both yourself and others in danger.

Once during my second year at university, my sister was coming to Reading to visit me. I had promised Olivia that I would pick her up from the station, so even though I was having some absences after a night out, I went to meet her at the station with my friend. I ended up in the hospital after having had a seizure alongside the canal in central Reading. I was far too close to the water when it happened. But I had made a commitment, and I hadn't wanted to let the epilepsy win, but in the end, it did.

During my time at university, I had many seizures. The mornings after a night out drinking would tend to be when I had a tonic-clonic seizure. I don't regret the decision to enjoy my time at

Reading, but I do wonder if my brain would be in a better condition if I had not been so determined to present as a young adult without health issues. What if I had accepted my epilepsy sooner?

I have experienced an Amsterdam hospital (probably the best), a French hospital, a German Hospital, and a few UK hospitals due to my epilepsy. Having an EHIC card enabled getting care in Europe to be possible and simple. It forever annoys me that travel insurance is more expensive to those like me with a pre-existing health condition, whatever the level of risk. Generally, if there is travel insurance included in a deal, like with a bank, it is of no benefit to me.

The sound of a paramedic bringing you around is both a familiar and terrifying sound. To me, it means I have had a seizure, but also that I am safe. I am so grateful to all those paramedics who have cared for me. Your care and calm are a huge comfort to both myself and those around me. However, I will say that your questions always make me feel stupid and make my brain work more than it wants to at the time!

Upon realising I have had a tonic-clonic seizure, a realisation that probably happens a few times after a seizure as I drift in and out of consciousness, I am generally overwhelmed by feelings: disappointment, embarrassment, and sadness. I am always disappointed that I have had another seizure, absolutely gutted that the epilepsy has won. The level of embarrassment depends on the situation, but is always there; did I wet myself, who witnessed it, the fact that someone is having to look after me, etc. Sadness comes due to many things: loss of self, loss of strength, loss to another seizure.

During this era, I couldn't go 3 months without having a tonic-clonic seizure. It was exhausting. I knew another one would eventually come; it was only a matter of time. Eventually, around the end of 2018, I decided to stop drinking after multiple recommendations from my doctors. This helped enormously. Along with a change in medication, the removal of alcohol allowed a bit more control over late nights and sleep efficiency. I felt tired when my brain or body naturally became tired, as opposed to pushing through with the help of alcohol. The day after drinking became more predictable, and though I may be tired from a late night, there was less chance of me having a tonic-clonic seizure. I was more likely to have a good night's sleep. My last seizure for a while was in January 2019.

2024-5 brought a whole medication change. Coming off Epesri (Ethosuximide) and Zonisamide, I was moving (back) onto Keppra (Levetiracetam) and Lamotrigine. This change impacted my life in many ways, but throughout the change, my brain struggled. I had increasingly more absence seizures and had to keep a closer eye on my energy levels by not overdoing things or overstimulating my brain.

Throughout this time, I have needed to adjust to a change in my energy levels. I used to be able to do long walks, socialise more, and have full days. Now, it is like my bucket of energy has a leak in it. Sometimes the leak is tiny, and so the bucket leaks slower, sometimes it is a big hole which empties the bucket far too quick. Every day, the size of the leak is different.

MY LATEST TONIC-CLONIC SEIZURE

After 6 years and 8 months, I had another tonic-clonic seizure. This was my first one being alone and coming around alone, and the first nocturnal one I have knowingly had. I say knowingly, as there are many nocturnal seizures that go unnoticed. But it is certainly not a common occurrence for me. However, my sister did remind me that at times they have occurred just as I am trying to sleep, to allow my brain to rest. Such as when my absences have been clustering and increasing in frequency, or just after I have had one tonic-clonic seizure. In these situations, I try to sleep, but it's potentially just too late. However, these tonic-clonic seizures have always been during the day.

Prior to this tonic-clonic seizure on 23rd September, I had been on a lovely road trip holiday to Italy with my parents. On return, we got back to Bristol and went to see a play at the Bristol Old Vic. I didn't quite notice just how tired I was after the play. I only realised I was really tired, that I had pushed my brain too far, as I headed home. As I walked home alone, leaving my family to go their own way, I started having very intense absences, increasing in frequency. Normally, when I have an absence seizure, my body continues to move and function as the absences are short. But, on this occasion, I would find myself in the middle of a road or pavement just standing still and momentarily forget what I was doing. I got pretty worried and just kept trying to focus on getting home; there wasn't much else to do. The absences increased, but I got home and was going straight to sleep. This would usually be the solution, but on this day, I just must have pushed my brain that bit too far.

It was scary, this tonic-clonic seizure. Over the last six and a half years, the longer the seizure-free gap became, I had in my mind that the next seizure I had may be fatal. My logic was that my body would need to have a seizure so bad that it would last longer, be more intense, and I wouldn't come back from it. There is a thing called SUDEP, which stands for the sudden unexpected death of a person with epilepsy. Though not very common, this occurs in about 1 in 1,000 people with epilepsy and has affected many people and families. Having generalised epilepsy, I am more at risk of this. SUDEP has become a fear of mine, but one that I try to keep at bay because what can I do to stop it other than try to manage my epilepsy? I am generally of the opinion that there is no point in worrying about the things we cannot control - as you have probably gauged by this point! Though this is not always easy to do.

After going to sleep that evening, feeling cold and jittery, I had my first nocturnal seizure that I know of. Normally, there is someone there when I come around. They have answers that I do not, like how many seizures I had and how long they lasted. Having been alone, I didn't have any of this information. All I knew was the rough time I had gone to sleep, and that post-seizure I messaged my family at 12.32 am to let them know I had had a tonic-clonic seizure. I had no idea what had happened in the two or so hours in between.

I came around after this tonic-clonic, having no idea where I was (I was at home in my bed). It took me a long time to slowly realise that this place was familiar to me and then longer again to know that it was my home. This phase, directly after a seizure, is called the "post-ictal" phase, where the brain is recovering and coming around. During this time, I slowly took in things like that my pillow had blood on it, and that my teeth hurt.

I could not move. As I realised the reason for this was that my muscles were exhausted, I came to the conclusion that I had had a tonic-clonic seizure. As I couldn't walk to the bathroom mirror, I used my phone to take a picture of myself so I could try to tell what had happened and where the blood was coming from. I had blood on my face, and it seemed that it had come from inside my cheek.

I must have ground my teeth so much that I had also sensitised my front teeth, chipping them a little and shoving my bottom ones forward so that they clashed and hurt when I closed my mouth. I notified my family that I had had a seizure, so they were aware, took some Clobazam, and went back to sleep.

I had to take the whole of the next day to sleep on and off. The following day, I was still exhausted. Eating hurt because of my teeth, so I needed to eat specific foods that didn't require much biting.

Six and a half years without a tonic-clonic seizure. I was so angry and frustrated that no matter how careful I had been all year, allowing my brain to rest and adjust to the medication changes, the epilepsy had won again.

The tonic-clonic clock had reset.

Less than 3 months later, I had another tonic-clonic seizure just like this. I had had a normal day, nothing too strenuous and whilst getting ready for bed, I started having increasingly frequent and intense absence seizures. Within an hour of going to sleep, I woke up confused and sore. As with my previous tonic-clonic seizure I had injured myself and had limited information about the seizure.

The clock resets once again.

RELATIONSHIPS

I didn't appreciate until really recently how little people knew about epilepsy. I suppose this awareness came as I opened up about it more. The most frequent question I get is whether flashing lights trigger me. No, I am not photosensitive; in fact, most people with epilepsy don't have this as a trigger. For me I am triggered by stress and tiredness, aggravated by overstimulation of my brain.

The impact it has on different types of relationships varies.

FAMILY

There is a lot to say on how my family has been with me throughout this journey, but I will keep it short. My family has helped me to have as "normal" a life as possible. I have never been treated differently or hovered over by them. I was never denied an experience because of my epilepsy. They supported me and are always there for me when I need them. I will always be grateful for the way my parents handled my diagnosis, encouraging me to have great life experiences and not letting myself be restricted by my epilepsy.

There is, of course, worry, but also trust and unquestioned, never-ending support, which has made this journey easier. I can always talk to them without explaining myself. They have never made me feel bad when I have to opt out of something, but supportive and just let me know that I am missed. I am very lucky to have such a family.

FRIENDSHIPS

At the start of my journey with epilepsy, I struggled with the idea of others knowing about my condition. The thought of losing control over who knew and when they knew became a source of deep concern for me.

I did not want to have epilepsy, so I refused to accept it. I wanted to live without its restrictions, and I didn't want to accept that epilepsy had much impact on my life.

I had to tell people on my own terms. If I heard that someone had divulged my personal diagnosis to someone else, I would be really upset. I remember getting angry with my mum for doing this when I heard her mention my epilepsy to others in conversation. Thankfully, she listened to me. With hindsight, I was overly sensitive here, but at the time, it was another thing out of my control, and I was so determined not to be defined by my epilepsy.

When I went to boarding school at 16, I told my close friends, but not many people. I was still only having absence seizures, something I could hide easily enough that it wasn't so necessary for many others to know. As I turned 18 and had my first tonic-clonic seizure in the middle of the school grounds, my condition became well-known. But as I was about to leave school, I saw no change in others' behaviour towards me.

Come university, I again only told my close friends or people who needed to know, but having had a few tonic-clonic seizures by then, the decision became more dictated by safety. I tried to make sure someone around me knew that I had epilepsy. I always tried to make it sound like nothing, to show that it wouldn't make me a burden as a friend. I very much lived the university experience, drinking alcohol throughout university and enjoying late nights out. This increased both types of seizure but enabled me to have the full university experience. I was a hockey captain with all the fantastic team nights out, and enjoyed the Union and clubs in town.

The mornings after nights out, I would be more likely to have seizures if I tried to function on insufficient sleep. These would be impossible to hide, and at the time, the pattern was an increasing cluster of absences followed by at least one tonic-clonic seizure.

My closest friends and flatmates became most aware of my epilepsy and its behaviour. They witnessed both seizure types, calling ambulances and staying with me. They have seen me at my most vulnerable - the moment my brain and body stop communicating when my brain malfunctions, and the post-ictal phase after I realise I have had a seizure. They have had to deal with seeing me having a tonic-clonic seizure, a period during which I am unconscious. This no doubt involves a level of panic or fear, then the distress of watching me have the seizure, ensuring I am safe, and helping me during and after the seizure. They have been there for the paramedics, answering their questions when they arrive, and made them cups of tea whilst they all wait for me to come around.

These friends have done so much for me over the years, and these friendships have only become closer. I am so lucky to have such amazing people in my life. To these people – thank you.

After university and entering the work life aged 23, my decision to tell people was still for safety purposes. I continued to tell people cautiously, fearing their judgement. Remaining in denial but trying to be slightly less irresponsible, managing my triggers where possible. However, I did not like to miss out on socialising if I could help it, so I still drank alcohol, I still had late nights, but I was just more aware of the impact and would often be aware that the next day may have to be a write off. I knew I could not push through a day on little sleep, and to stay committed to plans was no longer really possible if I didn't get much sleep. So, if I'd been out the night before, I had to reluctantly remove myself from an activity the next day. So perhaps I was aware but not quite so responsible by this point! Putting my health first has taken a long time, but true friends have been understanding of this. It goes against my nature to cancel plans, but I have had to go with what my body needs and ignore the rest. The times that I have "pushed through" in order to stick to a commitment often ended in having a seizure, and though they are an unpleasant experience for me, they are also definitely not fun for those around me.

I finally decided to stop drinking around 2019 and very quickly saw a reduction in my tonic-clonic seizures. Not drinking after it had been part of my social life was a tough journey. At the time, it wasn't as socially acceptable as it is today to not drink alcohol, and most bars and pubs had a limited selection of soft drinks on offer. It took friends (and me) a long time to adjust to my change in drinking habits - not being included on a round of beers, not getting drunk alongside people on a night out, not having the alcohol to keep tiredness from hitting me earlier in the night, etc. I'd get replies of "go on, just have one" or "don't be boring". I had to gain the social confidence to stick to my guns and join in the fun without the Dutch courage.

Not drinking may have impacted some friendships or some social inclusion. Drinking gives you more energy, encourages us to let go easier, but also, drunk people tend to be happier to be around other drunk people and people on a similar energy level. Perhaps they feel less judgment of drunken behaviour around others who are also drinking alcohol than from a sober person.

I remember coming across things I hadn't done sober yet, different "milestones". Going to parties and weddings by myself without drinking, karaoke with friends without the alcohol (a tough one!), and dating without the additional courage and buzz of an alcoholic drink. These experiences can feel daunting, but then once done, they become easier. We don't need alcohol; it is just a social habit we have become used to. It is about learning to have confidence in yourself. It is quite refreshing in many ways; you are more aware of whether you're really enjoying a situation, and your reactions are more genuine than if they were alcohol powered.

I love music, and I love a good dance. When drinking alcohol, if at a party, I could carry on talking throughout the night, or dance to any song (good or bad). Now, I feel my natural energy level. I can have great long conversations with people if it's genuinely flowing, and I can dance for hours if I am enjoying the music and company.

When it comes to drinking, I am not teetotal. I have always enjoyed flavours in both food and wine, and I don't restrict myself if there is an experience to be had. If there is a wedding, I may toast with champagne over water, though one glass would last me a long time. If someone has an interesting bottle of wine or whiskey (for example), I will have a taste of it, but not a whole glass. It is a balance, and I am much more aware of an immediate impact that drinking alcohol can have on me.

As I have become more open to talking about epilepsy, it sometimes comes up in conversation with people I have just met, if relevant. Sometimes I discover that that person also has epilepsy, sometimes I am asked many questions about my condition, sometimes it is just accepted, and the conversation moves on. I do find that explaining my epilepsy can at times be a bit exhausting, and it is hard to know how deep to go into the answers. It is a balance of sharing knowledge and not changing the tone of the conversation.

I once told a hairdresser that I wasn't feeling too well, so would need to be a bit quiet - "nothing to worry about, I just have epilepsy, and I currently have low energy". When she discovered that I lived alone, she asked if I was ever afraid of having a fit, hitting my head, and no one finding me. Though not said with malintent, and probably saying out loud what others have thought, it could have been phrased better or just kept to herself. I do not find this something worth being too concerned about; anyone can find themselves in a similar situation. I feel as though thoughts like this could restrict and control my life too much.

However, in order for me to live independently and as safe as possible, one route I have since gone down is having a wearable fall monitor. The monitor I have is a wrist fall monitor and senses a jerking motion. If sensed, it contacts the care line, they call my phone, and if I do not answer their call, they will call my emergency contact, and if not them, the emergency services.

Another monitor I may consider is one that connects to a bed for those who have sleep epilepsy. The Bristol council has been so helpful throughout the process of getting a monitor installed, a safety measure, just in case, that puts mine and others' minds at ease. Having a monitor helps me live independently. I am lucky to have a little support group who will come check on me if anything happens. True friends in life accept you for who you are, allow you to be yourself, support you, and understand if plans change.

There are many types of friendships, all of which are important and have impacted my life in different ways. The friendships I have that provide both parties with happiness, understanding, and support are the ones that are most important to me. These friends are not necessarily always present in location, but I know they are there for me. My closer friends are those that I am able to be my whole self with, be vulnerable with, talk about all aspects of my life, including my epilepsy. This is something I have learnt throughout this journey of life and epilepsy. I have managed to gain a fantastic support group in my friends and family, and I am incredibly appreciative of all of them.

INTIMATE RELATIONSHIPS

Romantic relationships are slightly different. Understanding, trust, and honesty are characteristics that I have really grown to hold in the highest regard. Although an important trait in any relationship, they have become more important since my memory started depleting. Because of this, I began to rely on those close to me to be my memory.

In a relationship, this vulnerability can hold you open to gaslighting. You need someone you can trust to be honest about a memory or an agreement that was made and not twist something in their favour. This is an experience I have had. Being pushed to try and remember something that has been distorted, being blamed for not remembering specifics when it is not my fault. Experiencing this sort of behaviour can really chip away at your confidence, and for me, it made me feel incompetent, weak, and put me in a frequent state of self-doubt. With my brain how it is, I have had to learn to let things go, believe the other person, and not argue or be frustrated around differences of memory. It is by no means easy to do! Letting things go in a relationship is hard, and if trust and honesty do not exist, you can lose yourself at the same time.

Understanding from a partner that you need more sleep, that you may need some time to process information, that you will be forgetful, and sometimes lack focus, is super important.

There needs to be an understanding that you will have times where you wake up and will not be able to function particularly well. The knowledge and understanding from your partner that they may have to carry on the day without you. Understanding and respecting each other's differences is important in all relationships, but especially in intimate ones. We are all different people, and those with epilepsy are not the only ones whose brains behave differently.

To my knowledge, my epilepsy has never directly influenced someone's decision on whether or not to date me. However, I've learned that when the idea of my epilepsy becomes a lived reality for a partner, it can start to affect the relationship.

I used to spend a lot of time worrying about when to tell someone that I had epilepsy. I'd let a relationship deepen before saying anything, and then spend days dreading the conversation, afraid of how they might judge me. This applies to friends as well as romantic relationships. It is always hard to discuss. How much information do I give them that will be enough but not scare them away?

Over time, talking about my epilepsy has become easier. The more I talk about it, the easier it has become to give a quick summary of my condition and then take the conversation from there. For a long time, it was always caveated with comments like "it's not that bad" and "I'm quite lucky really". However, comments like this can also dismiss your own feelings around having epilepsy, and I have learnt not to do it so much. The conversation was mainly about keeping the other person at ease whilst telling them that I had epilepsy. Trying to keep the assumptions and judgment to a minimum, and also trying to avoid being pitied. Most guys ask further questions; others don't.

On one date, however, I told him I didn't drink, and I was then repeatedly asked why I didn't drink. I eventually said that I have epilepsy. As we were walking from the bar to a table, he joked that I shouldn't sit on the wobbly stool at the table "just in case I had a fit". This was our first and last date!

In a romantic relationship, though the epilepsy itself may not be an issue, the impacts of having epilepsy have complicated or influenced a relationship moving forward. An example of this is the impact of not being able to drive. This in itself removes my independence in a way that I struggle with, but it also influences where I live. As much as I love the countryside, living in a disconnected village in the middle of nowhere is just not an option for me.

I need to have my independence and the ability to get myself from A to B and not always require someone to give me a lift. For me, it is important to live somewhere where I can get around on foot that also has good public transport options. This isn't only for my own independence, but if in the future I am lucky enough to have children, I would not want to feel stuck at home, unable to take them places.

Aside from the ability to drive, the need for me to be able to opt out of activities and manage my tiredness levels sometimes does not suit the other person's lifestyle. If they have envisioned having a consistently active lifestyle with their partner, always keeping busy and socialising, it is difficult to see how I would keep up. I need days to rest, I don't drink, and I have to know I can prioritize my health without disappointing anyone. I've always struggled to push aside the feeling that I'm letting people down. If someone reinforced that insecurity over and over, the relationship would become unhealthy.

As I have got older and have shared my experiences with epilepsy more, I have become more likely to open up about my epilepsy earlier on in a relationship. I may not get too serious and go into the weeds with it, but I feel that, as it is part of me, the other person should know. If they don't want someone because they have epilepsy, then simply put, I don't want them.

It hasn't always been the case, however. I used to wait until it was necessary to mention, or as a relationship became more serious. It is always a point of trepidation for me. No matter how comfortable I have become at talking about it, no one wants to be rejected for something they cannot change and did not sign up for.

Epilepsy and life experiences have altered my way of thinking when it comes to dating. I put myself and my needs higher than I used to and try not to blame myself for not being able to reach someone else's expectations.

I do feel that the impacts or side effects of having epilepsy can take their toll on a relationship. The impacts of having epilepsy can initially seem to be character traits, but they are symptoms of the wider condition and are hard to manage. Some people may have ideas about having a partner who can do everything and anything with them, drink with them, and constantly be super active. People with epilepsy may be able to do loads one week or day and nothing the next. We can commit to a plan, but also need people around us who understand that our health has to come first, and from time to time, plans may need to change. We have to be able to manage our epilepsy in whatever way is needed. We are not alone in this; many people have to manage their energy levels and capacity to be sociable. Those of us with epilepsy just can't push our brains too hard, as we can have potentially dangerous consequences.

WORK LIFE

I have had a few different jobs in my life so far, from part-time roles in retail and hospitality, to working as a nanny, moving to the Czech Republic to work in recruitment, and then heading into the Marketing world. I joined the corporate world, working in different departments, including Marketing, Marketing Operations, and Sales Operations, and worked my way up in them. I implemented different technologies, worked with different stakeholders, and managed different projects.

I say this not to delve into my CV but to show that it is possible for people with epilepsy to have a job, and a good one, with challenges that push them.

I am smart. I have a variety of interests, have always enjoyed learning new things, and have historically thrived when having a varied job description. However, at 33, I am currently having to go through a journey of accepting the increased impacts my epilepsy now has on both my life and my work life. I have had to further accept that I *am* disabled and try to discover what my rights are as a disabled person in the workplace.

I noticed a change in my brain around 2021. I had noticed a regression in my memory and my processing skills, and mentioned it to a doctor when participating in a research project for the epilepsy society in Chalfont St Peter's. This research was to compare brain activity of siblings - one with epilepsy and one without. My brother was my epilepsy-free sibling.

I had mentioned this concern about brain regression to the doctor, but the findings in the cognitive tests of the trial were not significant enough at the time to spark worry. Since mentioning this, I have both altered medications and experienced further regression of my brain power. Whether due to my medication, age, or the many seizures I have had over the years, we can only surmise. However, I cannot say I have seen much improvement from the changes to my medication.

Telling people at work that I have epilepsy has always been a tough decision. As in every other situation, I always fear judgment and discrimination. As I have become increasingly accepting of the condition I was born with, I find it easier to share. During interviews, I used to divulge this information at the final stage of interviews, when I was a solid candidate and was able to explain the potential impacts of my epilepsy further to my potential manager. This was due to safety and awareness - someone at work should always know about my epilepsy. Now, I would tell my employer from the get-go, as my epilepsy has become a more prominent part of me and I may require increased understanding and flexibility. This is in part due to the application processes, where they ask about health conditions; it is not something I would lie about.

My colleagues have never created an issue for me around my epilepsy. Over recent years, as I experienced daily impacts of having epilepsy, I became more open to sharing my diagnosis so people can be more understanding if I am slower or have an absence seizure on a call, for example. I am very happy to discuss my epilepsy with those who ask and have not knowingly been treated differently at work because of it. I feel that if someone receives this information negatively, both in work and out, it just reflects poorly on their character, and I try not to take it personally.

Most of the time, the response is either an encouraging "I had no idea!" or the curious, recurring "So... are you sensitive to bright lights?"

Unconscious bias will no doubt be in play somewhere along the line. For example, frustration over absences and changes to work behaviour. I have only received some misunderstanding, and at times this has turned into frustration and a "just get on with it" attitude. Many people can push through stress, tiredness, a sleepless night, and over-simulating environments, but in my experience with my epilepsy, this is never a good idea and often ends in multiple seizures - absence and tonic-clonic. I cannot "just get on with it", or I would - my health has to come first, and this thought that someone with epilepsy can just push past it can be ignorant and create an uninclusive, stressful, and pressured environment. Sometimes, frustration from others arises when someone does not understand my struggle with a task or project, whether in understanding it or carrying it out. This tends to push me to share the impact my epilepsy has had with a colleague. Other than having slow days, I can find it hard to understand and process a request. I can also find it hard to sufficiently communicate to others, like explaining or providing updates on a project. At times, this requires further patience and understanding from colleagues. Until someone is aware of your condition, they are bound to lack some understanding.

Epilepsy is not well understood, both by those with epilepsy in their life but mostly by those who do not have the condition. Most people presume it is set off by flashing lights. Although for some, they are correct, in most cases, there are other triggers, and triggers are only part of it. It is difficult to portray all the symptoms of epilepsy and how the condition can impact someone, other than having a seizure. Increased tiredness, the unpredictability of epilepsy, and the general fact that just because you don't have a seizure, epilepsy can still impact the day. It is a hidden disability for a reason, and just avoiding a seizure can be exhausting in itself.

Everyone with a disability is capable of contributing to a team, and though capabilities may change, support and understanding from others are key to discovering where each of us shine. It serves no one to make someone else feel incapable.

In 2022, I was internally promoted, starting a new role working with different technologies for the Marketing teams, alongside other projects, including creating training programs. I was able to do the role at the start, working with new technologies and coordinating with different stakeholders. My epilepsy had been, on the whole, manageable and did not impact my work life too much.

During 2023, I discovered that the different projects and sub-projects were proving difficult for my brain to handle. My role had also altered a little, with a bit more variety. My memory was becoming worse, and it became harder to process tasks and split my focus at the speed I once had.

I came to discuss this with my then manager at the back end of 2023, and it was decided that I would have an Occupational Health assessment done. I had three conversations with occupational health throughout 2024 and 2025, all stating in summary that my health concerns, and the concerns of the company, were due to my epilepsy. It was around this time that I was starting my medication change, and so I had hope that my brain would improve.

I worked for my previous company for 7 years and 4 months. With this medication change, and the impact that having epilepsy has had on me, my work capabilities have changed. I eventually had to go off on a prolonged absence during my medication change, which ended up lasting months. I was not able to work full-time, needed much more sleep, and saw that managing work and my health was impacting my ability to cope with life. I was struggling. At the same time, I was grappling with the unknown—wondering whether my brain had changed for good or if it was just the lingering effects of my medication. It's an emotional journey to accept that the worst-case scenario may be the case - that these changes were indeed permanent. This also comes with grieving old memories and previous capabilities. Throughout this medication change process, I was very clear with my employers about the journey into the unknown. I was candid with them, sharing all I knew about the situation, and exposing my vulnerability in order to provide some clarity. Because the brain remains largely unknown—and because everyone's body responds differently—I rarely had any clear answers to offer my employer. I did not have a broken arm that will roughly be better in 8 weeks; I have a faulty brain, which impacts the whole body and is unpredictable to both me and the neurologists. It is therefore hard to provide clear answers on helpful adjustments or my recovery timeline. It also became hard to confidently stand up for myself when I know my brain isn't functioning at full strength. I know that I was previously capable of more, I just do not know what I am fully capable of right now, or whether I will remain on reduced ability for good.

I found my then employers to be superficially understanding, as is potentially to be expected, both because I used to be capable of more and because they are not the sufferers of this condition. This superficial understanding became a bit of a shock when it came down to formal meetings. I did not feel understood or supported in the long run, only during initial one-to-one meetings, before they showed their frustration during my sick leave. Whilst I wish I were not in a health limbo, knew my capabilities, and had all the answers, I have to try not to let it get to me or stress me out too much because this is, of course, one of my triggers. I do let myself be angry and frustrated now and then, as it isn't healthy to keep it in, but then I have to let it go and move on.

I was recently let go on the grounds of capability, whilst off sick, which has not sat right with me. The reasoning (my current capability) and the occupational health assessments are all intrinsically linked to my epilepsy and my medication change. Using grey areas of law makes it easy for companies to get away with treating disabled people poorly, especially those with hidden disabilities.

ACCEPTANCE

The more I have talked about epilepsy, the easier it has become. I had to learn to accept that certain things were out of my control; my loss of memory and forgetfulness, not being able to rely on being well every day, having a lower energy level - the list goes on. I try to focus on my core priorities and what I can control; they are easier to manage.

When telling a story, I have learned to accept that I sometimes cannot remember certain parts and try not to get too hung up on the words and facts that I forget. I try to push on with the story regardless - unless there are just too many missing pieces! I have had to learn to forgive myself and give myself a break.

Acceptance has not only come through talking about it but also seeing first-hand how little it is understood. It has come through having to explain it to so many people and experiencing the impact it is now having on my life.

Joining Facebook groups and working with epilepsy charities to share my story alongside others has shown me that I am not alone in my experience. I am part of a research panel for parents and patients, which has given me a space to share my experiences with epilepsy. I can then hopefully have a positive impact on the experience of many more people who will be diagnosed with epilepsy in the future.

Deciding not to drink was a large step towards accepting that I have this lifelong condition. I had to let go of the hope that my brain would grow out of it, and I had to make a sensible decision.

Staying committed to this decision helped me further along the road to accepting this part of me that I did not choose.

Accepting that I will probably never be able to drive has been tough, but also a relief. It has enabled me to make more life decisions, removing the hypothetical as an option. I live somewhere that I love, where I can get around by myself, access public transport, and do things that I need and want to do, like meeting friends, going to the dentist, or seeing a play. Even if there were a point in my life where I could drive, I would always have the fear and anxiety of having another seizure and having my freedom removed. Having another seizure will always remain a possibility, and I have decided not to put myself in the position where I lose my independence. Public transport in the UK is not consistent or reliable. I often rely on friends as chauffeurs to get around places that are out of town and don't have a train station. This is more of a necessity if I am out in the countryside.

Acceptance has enabled me to put my health first. I allow myself the space I need to recuperate. I pre-empt a situation of not being well enough to commit to a plan. Having a backup where I am not stuck somewhere feeling unwell removes a certain amount of anxiety. I will let myself slip away from an event early.

Acceptance goes a long way to remove the guilt, shame, and sadness that can come with letting people down, missing out, or feeling like a burden.

Acceptance is a form of self-love and self-care, helping to reduce the anxiety, stress, and fear of a situation. Whatever the outcome, it will be okay.

BECOMING AN ARTIST

I wanted to find a calming, creative outlet that contrasted with my last job and gave me time away from technology. I decided to give painting a go, something I had never really taken to at school. At school, I felt the pressure of perfection and restriction of style. But as an adult, removing the restriction, I have fallen in love with it.

I bought some acrylics and got started. I loved it! The freedom it allowed, the lack of restriction, the creativity it unlocked.

Painting is liberating and enables self-expression. I find the process therapeutic and calming for my brain. It is a world that is mine that I dictate and feel competent at, a feeling that was removed during my previous full-time role. Even when I am having a bad day, where I don't trust myself to leave the house and interact with people, I can sit, listen to music, and paint. A crappy day can be instead one lost in creative productivity.

Painting and drawing remained a hobby. I grew in skill, enjoying the learning experience of challenging myself and trying out new materials. Learning and being inspired by other artists also grew my confidence and opened me up to this new world. I ended up exhibiting my work both online and in venues. This world has made me feel capable, has given me flexibility that suits my brain, and provides me a calm space to relax. Creating art helps me to process emotions, express myself, and share my views. I had found the outlet I was looking for and more.

When I was let go from my job in August 2025, I remained unwell. I was still changing my medication and feeling the impact of it. My confidence in my abilities had been highly diminished, and I was not in a space to apply for any new jobs. Not only had I been made to feel incapable, but I also did not know how my brain would be after finishing my medication change. Would it be "back to normal" or is this it for the foreseeable? We had no answers yet; it remained a wait-and-see situation.

I had to remember to be kind to myself and give myself some space to get better. So I chose to make a go of being an artist, a full-time artist and see if it was sustainable. It was a major change and a leap I was somewhat pushed into, and an even bigger adjustment to navigate! But after the way work had been, I felt an enormous relief to be able to do something that both suited my health and allowed me to focus on something I really loved. I could spend my time feeling capable.

Being an artist allows me the flexibility to work with my disability. Not having a set schedule allows me to give my brain space to recover and relax when it's needed. My week's structure can adapt to my brain. I can be creating on some days, both art and social content. On other days, I can do admin, applications, and strategy. Leaving the remaining days to absorb culture and nature. I absolutely love this world I have created. My journey with epilepsy hugely influences and inspires my artwork. My loss of memory, my struggle to get words out, vulnerability, and letting go are core themes to a lot of my work. Processing my feelings around my epilepsy through paint continues to be a healing and liberating process. A therapist once told me that it would be great to delve into the impact my epilepsy has had on me. I had never before considered that I had been much impacted by this journey with epilepsy, but of course I had! It requires a constant re-evaluation of my life. Painting it out has been an amazing way to process this journey. I have included some of my epilepsy inspired pieces in this book.

Though I may have to eventually subsidise being an artist with a part-time role, for now, it brings me so much joy.

LIVING WITH, NOT AGAINST EPILEPSY

Life with epilepsy has been an ever-changing journey - which has had its low points! But it's a journey where I have discovered so much about myself and my brain. I have learned what is truly important to me and what I should prioritise in life. It has taken me years to process the changes, to learn and adapt. The journey continues to be a tough and capricious one, and although it has impacted many aspects of my life, I refuse to let the epilepsy take over.

The support of my family and friends has helped and encouraged this determination. They have helped me to experience life to its fullest and have always been there for me when needed. This support system has enabled me to feel capable and included. With this support, I have travelled a lot, lived abroad, played a lot of sports, flown a glider, been horse riding, had relationships, worked and had promotions, had a great social life, had great nights out, and much more. I try not to make restrictions that I am not happy with, but I do listen to my body's limits. Any restrictions I have made, like removing alcohol, I have done so at a time I was ready. Remember, those of us with epilepsy are not alone in having to adjust our lives as we get older, pushing our limits just has bigger, more potentially dangerous consequences.

I hope that sharing my journey allows those with epilepsy or perhaps another life-changing condition to see that they are not alone in how they feel. Perhaps they can even take on some of the things that I have learnt along the way and use them to help their lives feel more manageable. For those without epilepsy, I hope that sharing my journey so far has opened your eyes to the wider impact of epilepsy.

I continue to learn and adjust to the hand I have been dealt and see the positives where I can.

Thank you so much for reading this book, it means a lot to me that you have taken the time to understand more about a life with epilepsy.

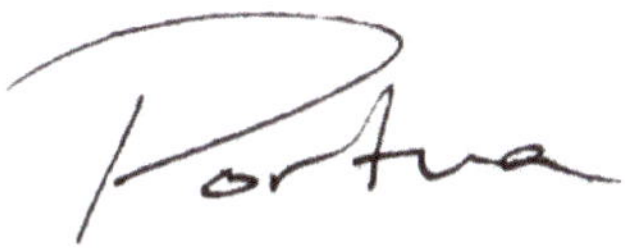

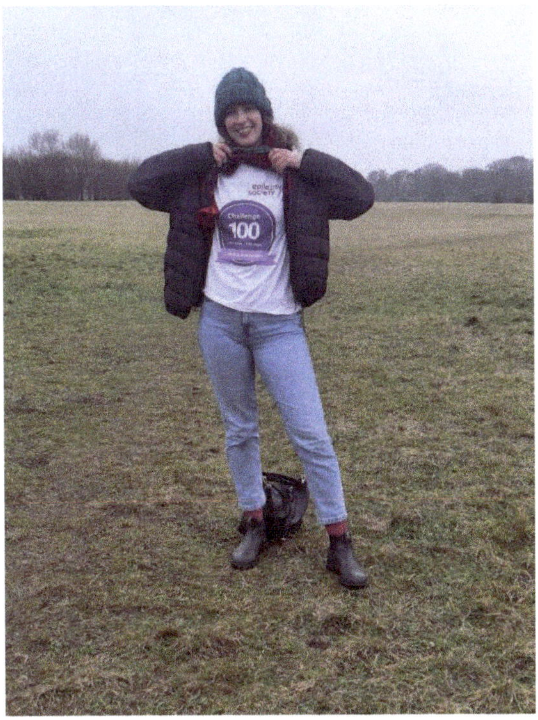

ART FROM PORTIA

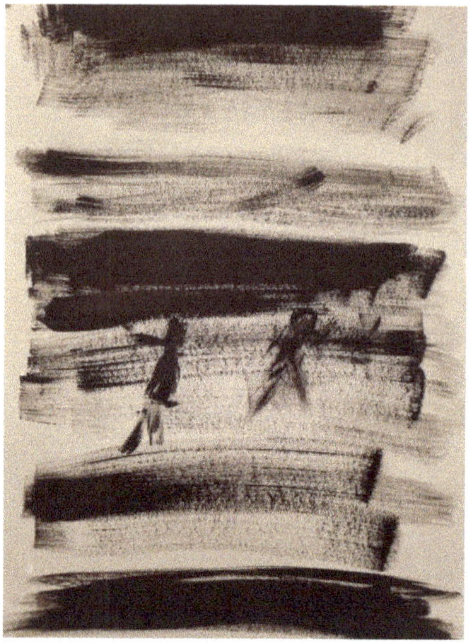

"Through the Fog"

This painting portrays how it feels trying to function on a slightly bad day. Even without a seizure, the day can be a struggle, and you can feel removed from the world.

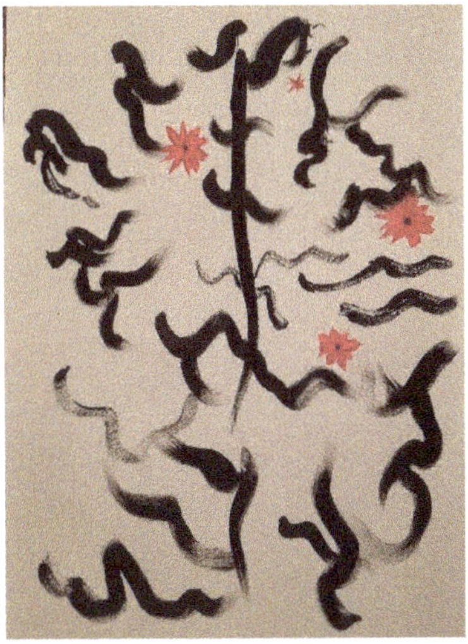

"Fireworks"

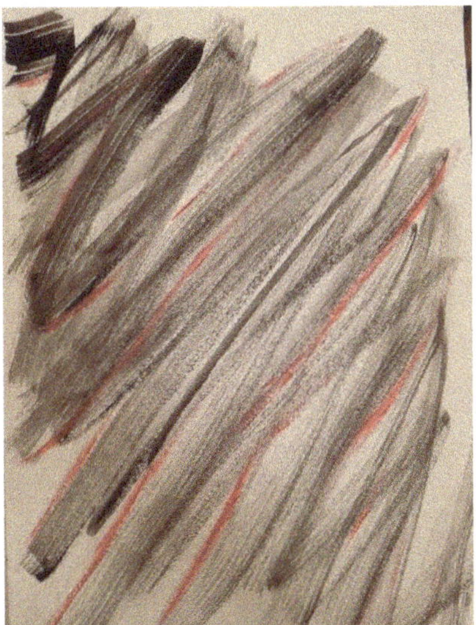

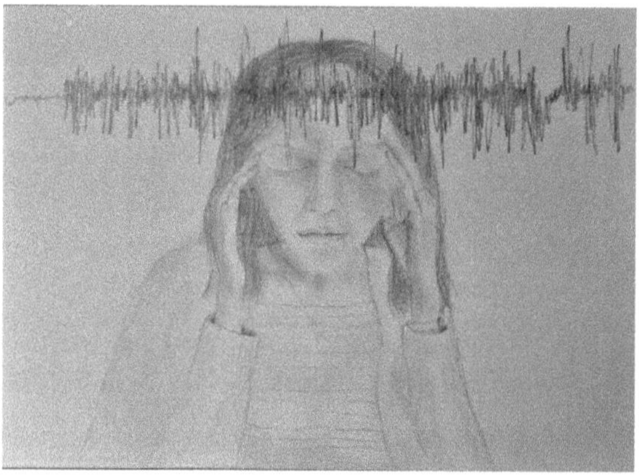

"Not Free"

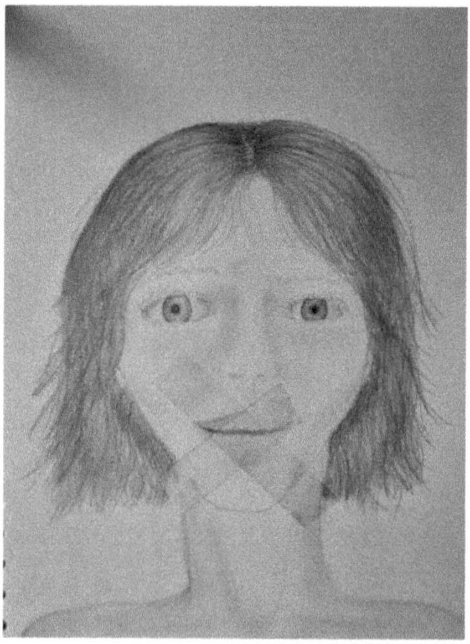

This one is a sketch showing the voice that is sometimes taken away. The struggle to speak because of a lack of energy, difficulty processing and following the conversation, or because the memory is failing you.

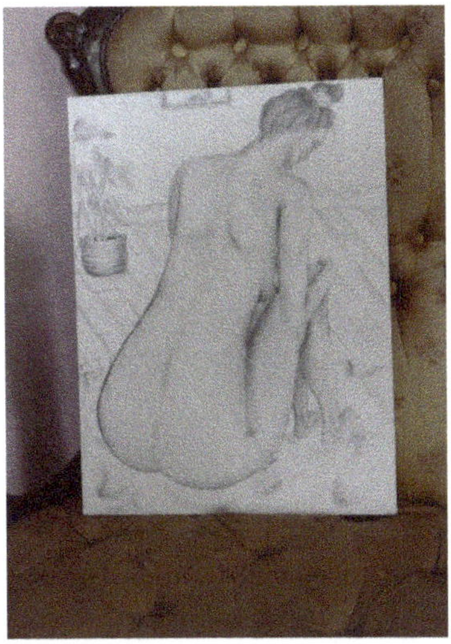

"Vulnerability"

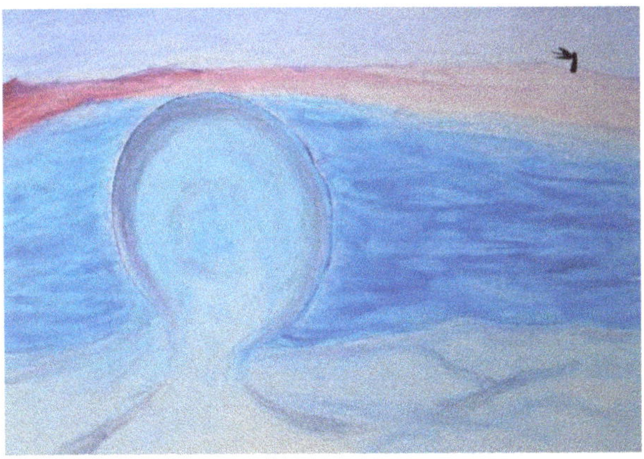

"Memories"

The painting reflects the ebb and flow of memory—some moments sharp and vivid, others fading quietly into the background. It captures the quiet grief of saying goodbye to what we can no longer hold onto.

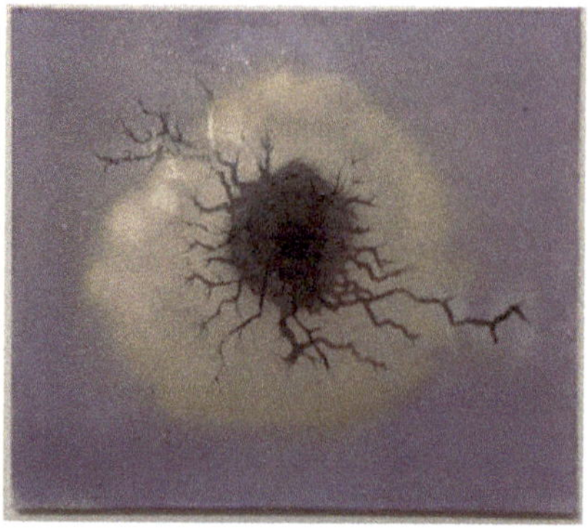

"Unwanted Activity"

Purple for the brain and for all of us living with epilepsy. Gold for our strength, our resilience, our hope...and the medication that helps us navigate each day. Black for the seizures that arrive uninvited - the unwanted activity that interrupts our lives but will never define us.

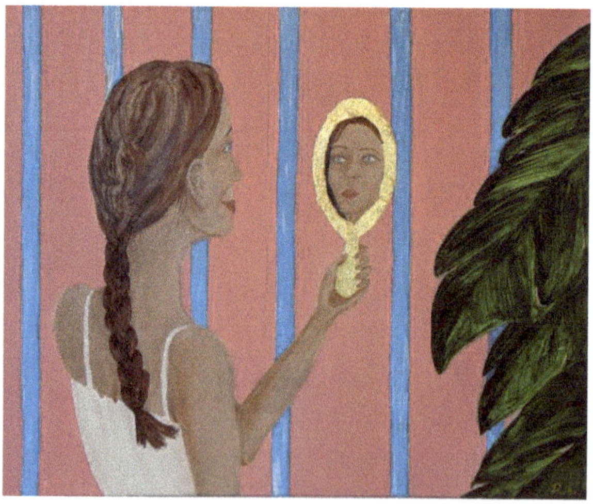

"Beneath the Smile" shows the face we put on for others; the mask society pushes us to wear when inside we are crying.

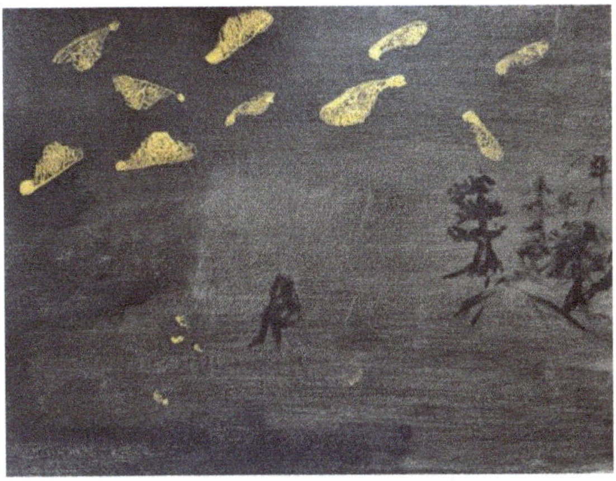

"Opportunities" - Though not all opportunities are available to you, there is always another opportunity around the corner.

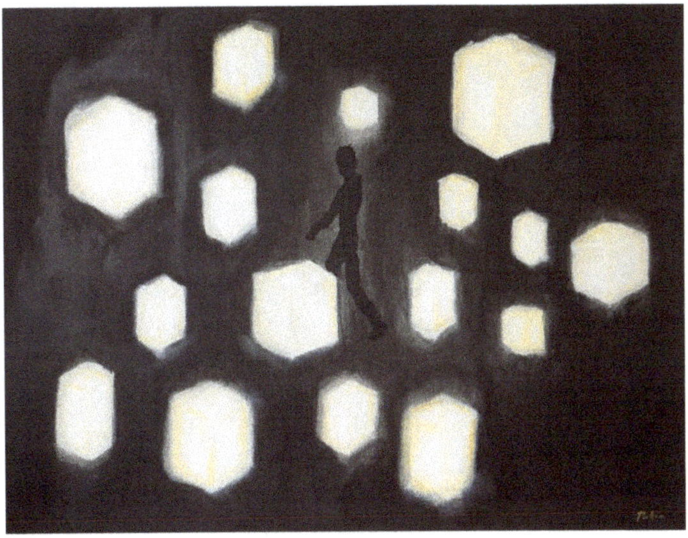

"There's Always Light"

Life is made up of good and bad - memories, experiences, and influences. Let the light of the good illuminate the darkness. You are not alone in your struggles and are surrounded by light - you just need to let it in.

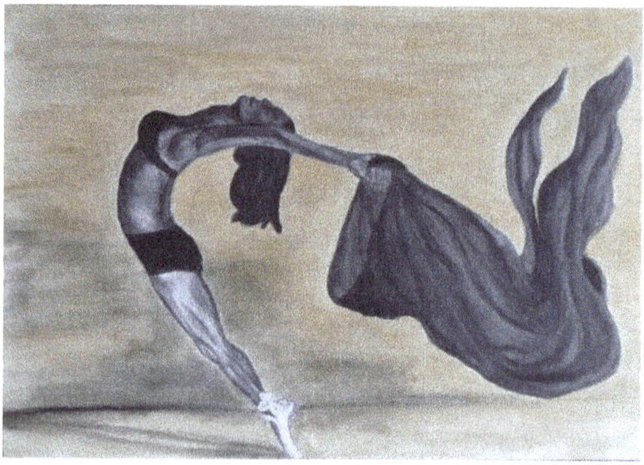

"Letting Go"

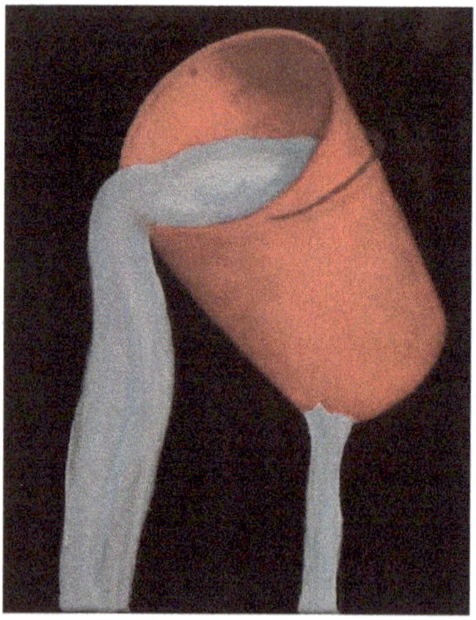

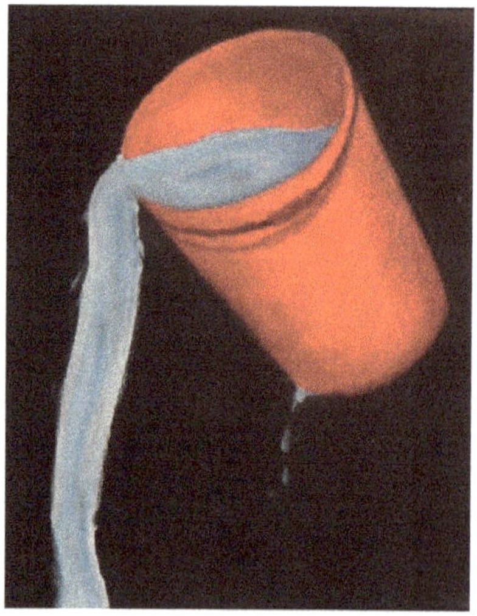

My energy comes in a bucket...with a leak.

Some days it drips.

Some days it pours out.

Every day, it's different.

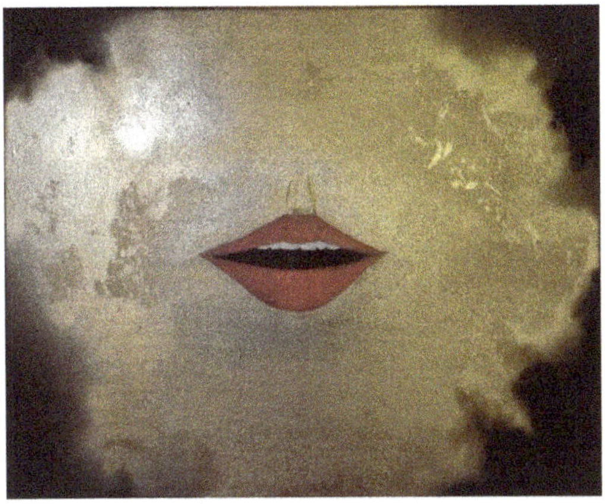

"Whispers of Gold"

The quiet strength of the human voice. These lips carry words that shimmer with the power to inspire, heal, and transform. Even the softest whisper can leave a golden imprint on the world.

The message of this painting goes hand in hand with my reasons behind writing this book. Sharing our stories helps others know that they are not alone, and in just that, the world feels lighter.

AUTHOR'S BIO

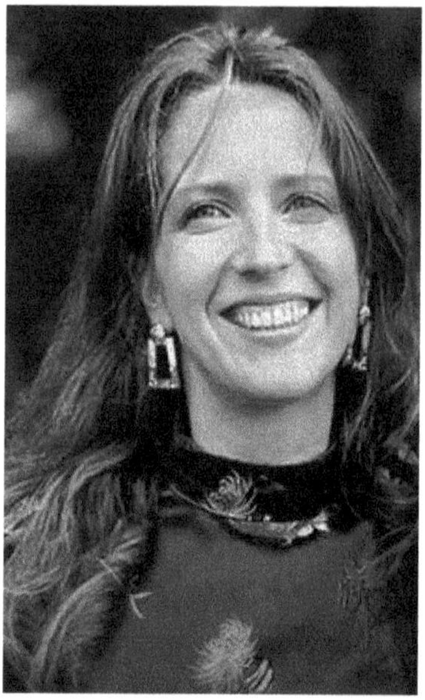

Portia Hibbert is a Bristol-based writer whose debut autobiographical book draws on over twenty years of lived experience with epilepsy. Diagnosed at thirteen, she has long navigated the challenges of the condition, and through this book, she shares a story shaped by resilience, creativity, and self-discovery. Through sharing these experiences, Portia hopes to raise awareness and improve understanding of epilepsy. Alongside writing, she has recently embraced painting as a creative outlet, discovering a more balanced way of life that supports both her health and artistic expression.

www.artfromportia.com

@artfromportia

One in 100 people in the UK has epilepsy.

Be accepting, be understanding, and be aware.

What Should You Do If You Witness Someone Having A Seizure?

Calm

Time

Cushion

Call

Calm - stay calm and be a calming voice.

Time - time the seizure or check the time so you can know how long the seizure lasts. This is important - the longer it lasts, the higher the risk to the person.

Protect - Only move the person if they are in a dangerous place (i.e., the road), move objects from around them that they may hit themselves on.

Cushion - cushion their head with a jumper or something to hand so they don't hit their head.

Do not restrict them or put something in their mouth - allow the seizure to happen.

Check for any medical jewellery or ID

Give them space – do not crowd them.

After The Seizure:

- Recovery position - roll them into the recovery position.
- Reduce embarrassment – they may have lost bladder control, cover this if possible.
- Stay with them and calmly reassure them.

Call an ambulance if:

- it is their first seizure
- if the seizure lasts more than 5 minutes
- if they have another seizure without recovery in between

Helpful Resources

I thoroughly suggest taking a look at Epilepsy Action UK and Epilepsy Society. Both charities have great resources and support.

These suggested resources are targeted towards UK patients, mentioning health services that may not exist in other countries. Much of the advice may be applicable worldwide, but please be aware that care options will vary country to country.

www.ingramcontent.com/pod-product-compliance
Lightning Source LLC
Chambersburg PA
CBHW040827150926
51501CB00050B/1637
9781807043728